ESSENTIAL GUIDE TO ROSACEA

Understanding, Managing, and Thriving: The Comprehensive Guide to Rosacea

DR. CASEY LOREN

DISCLAIMER

This book's content is only meant to be used for general informative purposes. Although the author has taken great care to ensure the content is accurate and thorough, no warranties or assurances on the information's accuracy, correctness, or reliability are provided. It is recommended that readers employ their own judgment and discretion when applying any material found in this book to their particular situation.

The information in this book is not intended to replace professional advice, nor is the author an expert in any of the subjects covered. It is recommended that readers consult with experienced professionals regarding any particular issues or concerns.

Any name that may be mentioned or referred in this book does not imply endorsement, recommendation, or relationship on the part of the author with any person, entity, good, website, or association. These references are made only for informational purposes and are not meant to be taken as recommendations or endorsements.

The information contained in this book may cause readers to suffer loss or damage, for which the author disclaims all obligation and accountability. The only people accountable for the decisions and actions taken by readers using the information presented are themselves.

Any names, characters, companies, locations, activities, occasions, and incidents referenced in this book are either made up or the result of the author's imagination. Any likeness to real people, living or dead, or to real things is entirely coincidental.

This book's content may change at any time, without prior notice, according to the author. The onus is on the reader to verify whether there have been any updates or revisions.

The reader accepts the conditions of this disclaimer by reading this book. Please do not

read this book or use its contents if you do not
agree to these terms.

CHAPTER 1

ROSACEA: A BASIC OVERVIEW

Rosacea: A Medical Term

Rosacea is an inflammatory skin disorder that mostly manifests on the face and can lead to redness, pimples, visible blood vessels, and even irritation of the eyes in certain individuals. A gradual onset is typical, beginning with reddening and flushing of the cheeks, nose, forehead, and chin that continues throughout the day.

Rosacea Varieties and Subtypes

Rosacea can be classified into four basic types:

1. Characteristics of erythematotelangiectatic rosacea include flushing of the face and the presence of visible blood vessels.

2. In papulopustular rosacea, red lumps (papules) and pustules (pimples) fill the skin and resemble acne.

3. Skin thickening, specifically on the nose (rhinophyma) but also on the chin, forehead, and ears, is a symptom of phymatous rosacea.

4. Dryness, inflammation, redness, and even blurred vision can be symptoms of ocular rosacea.

What Causes Rosacea and What Sets It Off

No one knows for sure what causes rosacea, however, several things can bring it on or make it worse:

1. Rosacea tends to run in families, so knowing someone with the condition can make you more likely to get it yourself.

2. Mites of the Demodex species: These microscopic skin parasites may have a role in inducing inflammation.

3. Facial redness and flushing might be caused by overactive vascular response or anomalies in blood vessels.

4. Factors in the Environment: Sunlight, spicy meals and drinks, alcohol, stress, and several skin care products are common environmental triggers.

Signs and symptoms

Rosacea symptoms might differ from person to person, but often include:

1. Ongoing flushing of the face

2. Easily flushed and reddening

3. Telangiectasia, or blood vessels that are visible

4. Mild pimples that look like acne

5. The skin becomes thicker, particularly around the nose

6. Redness, dryness, and inflammation of the eyes (ocular symptoms)

Medical Evaluation and Diagnosis

A dermatologist or ophthalmologist usually does a comprehensive skin and ocular exam to diagnose rosacea. Medical evaluations might involve:

1. By looking at the skin, we can detect telltale symptoms including redness, pimples, and visible blood vessels.

2. The purpose of a skin biopsy is to diagnose a specific condition by removing a little piece of skin for testing in a lab.

3. Examining the eyes for symptoms of ocular rosacea, which may include using specific dyes to identify inflammation, is part of a comprehensive eye checkup.

Rosacea and Acne: The Essential Distinctions

Although there may be some overlap in symptoms, rosacea and acne are quite separate conditions:

1. Compared to acne's comedones (blackheads and whiteheads), papules, and pustules, rosacea is more likely to cause facial redness, flushing, and visible blood vessels.

2. In addition to the more common acne-related symptoms, rosacea can cause ocular issues such as dryness and inflammation of the eyes.

3. Additionally, rosacea often affects adults over the age of 30 and acne typically occurs during adolescence, while the lesions of each condition manifest at different ages and in different places.

Popular Fallacies Regarding Rosacea

Rosacea is often misunderstood, and here are a few examples:

1. Although rosacea is primarily a skin disorder, it can also manifest in the eyes (ocular rosacea) and cause considerable pain and issues with vision.

2. Although proper skincare routines do help, rosacea is not an indication of uncleanliness.

3. Though it has certain symptoms with acne, rosacea is its skin ailment with its own set of causes and methods of treatment.

Rosacea and Its Effects on Daily Living

Physical and mental well-being can both take a hit when dealing with rosacea. Feelings of inadequacy, shame, and social anxiety may accompany rosacea's visual symptoms. Also, ocular rosacea can cause dry eyes, pain, and vision problems, which can make it hard to go about your day-to-day business.

Factors Contributing to Epidemiology

Millions of people around the world suffer from rosacea, which is more common among persons of fair complexion who are of Northern European origin. Although men can have more severe cases, women are more likely to be afflicted. Fair skin, a family history of rosacea, and exposure to sun and spicy meals are some of the environmental triggers that can cause the condition.

State of the Art and Recent Developments in Rosacea Research

Rosacea research is ongoing with the goals of improving diagnostic tools, developing more effective treatments, and understanding the underlying causes of the condition. New developments encompass:

1. Research into how the skin microbiome and Demodex mites contribute to the onset of rosacea.

2. The creation of specific medications to treat skin barrier failure, vascular anomalies, and inflammation.

3. Determining the extent of disease and the efficacy of treatment through the investigation of non-invasive imaging methods.

4. Research studies testing new treatments for rosacea, including oral drugs, topical formulations, and combinations of these.

All things considered, rosacea sufferers have reason to be optimistic about the future of treatment thanks to ongoing research.

CHAPTER 2

ROSACEA: A PHYSIOLOGICAL STUDY

Skin Structure and Function

To fully grasp rosacea, one must be well-versed in the anatomy of the skin. Multiple layers make up the skin; the epidermis is the outermost, followed by the dermis and subcutaneous tissue. The protective and homeostasis-preserving functions of each layer are interdependent. In contrast to the protective epidermis, which lies just below the skin's surface, the dermis houses the body's vital organs, including blood vessels, nerves, hair follicles, and sweat glands. The face, and the central region in particular, can be affected by rosacea, which can cause redness, irritation, and the appearance of visible blood vessels as a result of several different triggers.

How Blood Vessels Contribute to Rosacea

The pathophysiology of rosacea is heavily influenced by blood vessels, particularly telangiectasia (visible blood vessels) and flushing. Rosacea is characterized by an increased sensitivity to environmental triggers and a chronic reddening of the face as a result of dilated blood vessels. Treatments for rosacea frequently focus on this vascular component to alleviate redness and other symptoms.

Rosacea Inflammatory Routes

Rosacea is characterized by inflammation, which further contributes to the appearance of papules, pustules, and erythema. In response to certain stimuli, the immune system secretes inflammatory mediators such as cytokines and chemokines. These mediators increase the inflammatory response, recruit more immune cells, and widen blood vessels. To manage rosacea and stop the illness from getting worse, it is essential to target these pathways.

Rosacea + Demodex Mites

Rosacea has been linked to Demodex mites, specifically Demodex folliculorum and Demodex brevis. Although these tiny mites are common on healthy skin, rosacea sufferers may experience an overabundance of them, which could lead to an inflammatory reaction and an immune system response. Topical medicines that target mite populations are one potential therapy strategy that could be informed by a better understanding of Demodex's function in rosacea.

Rosacea and Hereditary Factors

There is some evidence of familial clustering of rosacea cases, suggesting a genetic component to the disease's susceptibility. Rosacea susceptibility may be influenced by variations in genes that are involved in immunological function, skin barrier integrity, and vascular control. The intricate interaction between hereditary predisposition and environmental triggers is illustrated by the fact that environmental factors and triggers also have a substantial impact on disease presentation in rosacea.

The Role of the Immune System

Both the innate and adaptive immune responses have a role in the development of rosacea, which is an intricate immunological-mediated illness. The rosacea-specific dysregulation of immune pathways can cause hypersensitivity reactions, vascular permeability, and tissue damage. One of the most important aspects of managing rosacea and reducing symptom flare-ups is modulating immunological responses.

Disruption of Neurovascular Function

The irregular connections between the neurological system and blood vessels, known as neurovascular dysregulation, can amplify the symptoms of rosacea. Patients with rosacea may experience redness and flushing of the face as a result of increased blood flow and vasodilation brought on by nerve signals. The management of rosacea-related vascular symptoms requires an understanding of neurovascular dysregulation and the targeting of this condition.

Skin Reactions to Common Triggers

The first step in managing rosacea is to identify potential triggers and stay away from them. Certain skincare products, sun exposure, hot drinks, spicy foods, alcohol, and stress are common triggers. Rosacea symptoms can be worsened and flare-ups can occur when these factors cause vasodilation, inflammation, or neurovascular reactions. Patients must be educated about trigger avoidance to maintain skin health and effectively treat their illness.

The Importance of Sunlight

For many people who suffer from rosacea, being in the sun is the worst possible scenario. Skin inflammation, blood vessel damage, and worsening of redness and flushing can all be caused by exposure to ultraviolet (UV) radiation. Sunscreen, hats, and shade are musts for rosacea sufferers who want to keep their skin safe from UV rays and reduce the frequency and severity of flare-ups.

The Role of Hormones in Rosacea

Rosacea symptoms can be influenced by hormonal factors, especially in women. A worsening or recurrence of rosacea symptoms may occur at the same time as a hormonal shift, such as during menstruation, pregnancy, or menopause. Hormonal variables have a role in the pathogenesis of rosacea by influencing vascular tone, immunological responses, and the function of the skin barrier. Rosacea symptoms may be better managed with lifestyle changes or medication that reduces hormonal swings.

Both healthcare providers and patients can benefit from a better understanding of the physiology and triggers of rosacea to create individualized strategies for effective therapy. To get the best results in managing rosacea, it is necessary to address the intricate relationship between skin structure, vascular function, immunological responses, and environmental factors.

CHAPTER 3

ROSACEA TREATMENT OPTIONS

Products for External Use: Lotions, Creams, and Gels

A lot of people who suffer from rosacea start by using topical treatments. Metronidazole, azelaic acid, and sulfur are common components found in these topical medications, which are available in a variety of formulations such as creams, gels, and lotions. The redness, irritation, and rosacea-related papules and pustules can be managed with the use of these products. For optimal results and to reduce the likelihood of side effects like dryness or irritation, it is crucial to apply the product according to your dermatologist's instructions.

Antibiotics and anti-inflammatory medications are taken orally.

Oral medication may be recommended for rosacea in more severe instances or if topical therapies don't work. To alleviate inflammation and regulate bacterial development on the skin, antibiotics like doxycycline or minocycline can be helpful. To temporarily ease flare-ups, anti-inflammatory medications such as low-dose oral corticosteroids may also be prescribed. To keep an eye on how well these drugs are working and for any unwanted side effects, it is essential to take them precisely as directed and to schedule frequent checkups with your doctor.

Treatments with Lasers and Light

The use of light and lasers to target blood vessels and diminish redness has completely transformed the way rosacea is treated. Pulsed dye lasers (PDL) and intense pulsed light (IPL) therapy are two methods that can improve the look of skin by reducing the visibility of blood vessels. To achieve the best results, these treatments are usually performed in the office of a dermatologist and may involve more than one session. Despite its typically low risk, therapy may cause some short-lived side effects, such as redness or swelling.

A Chemical Peel with Dermabrasion

Dermabrasion and chemical peels may be suggested for rosacea patients whose skin has thickened or developed textural problems. Chemical peels employ chemicals to exfoliate and renew the skin, whereas dermabrasion removes the outer layer of skin using a revolving brush or tool with diamond tips. To minimize risks and maximize intended outcomes, these procedures should only be conducted by those with the necessary training.

Skin Care Products and Sunscreens

To control rosacea, you must use the right skincare products. To lessen dryness and sensitivity, use a moisturizer containing calming components like hyaluronic acid or ceramides. These will help hydrate and fortify the skin's barrier. Protect yourself from the sun's rays, which can bring on rosacea flare-ups, by using an SPF 30 sunscreen or higher. Avoid further aggravation by searching for fragrance-free, non-comedogenic products.

A Change in Diet and Lifestyle

Hot drinks, spicy foods, alcohol, and very hot or cold weather are some of the lifestyle factors that can make rosacea symptoms worse. Skin conditions can be greatly improved by making dietary modifications and avoiding triggers. To further reduce the likelihood of irritation and inflammation, it is recommended to follow healthy skincare practices such as using mild cleansers and staying away from harsh chemicals.

Methods for Dealing with Stress

Mindfulness, meditation, yoga, or deep breathing exercises are great ways to reduce stress, which is a typical cause of rosacea flare-ups. A decrease in systemic inflammation and an improvement in skin health can result from learning to relax and unwind.

Alternative Medicine and Domestic Hygiene

Green tea extract, aloe vera gel, and oatmeal masks are some of the natural therapies that some people use to alleviate the symptoms of rosacea. Natural treatments can still trigger reactions in sensitive skin, so it's important to talk to a dermatologist before attempting any new treatment, even though these alternatives may help soothe the skin.

Additional Treatment Options: Meditation, Acupuncture

In addition to conventional rosacea treatments, alternative medicine practices like acupuncture and meditation can help alleviate symptoms and improve general health. Although they might not alleviate rosacea symptoms in and of themselves, they can help with a more comprehensive strategy for controlling the illness.

Novel and Investigated Treatments

Innovative medicines such as microbiome-based treatments, peptide-based drugs, and targeted immunotherapies are among the new rosacea therapy approaches that are the subject of ongoing research. These methods may provide patients with more tailored and efficient choices for managing their rosacea in the future, although they are currently in the testing phase. If you are thinking about trying any new therapy, you should talk to your doctor first.

People with rosacea can benefit greatly from being well-informed about their treatment options. This will allow them to collaborate closely with their healthcare professionals to create unique treatment regimens that target their symptoms, triggers, and lifestyle variables. Rosacea can be properly managed and overall skin health and quality of life can be improved with a combination of medicinal therapies, skincare practices, and lifestyle alterations.

CHAPTER 4

FORMULATING AN INDIVIDUALISED STRATEGY FOR THE CONTROL OF ROSACEA

Collaborating with a Skin Surgeon

An important ally in the fight against rosacea is a dermatologist. They can precisely identify your illness, evaluate its seriousness, and design an individualized treatment strategy. Make sure to go into depth about your symptoms, treatments you've tried in the past, and product reactions throughout your appointments. Your dermatologist can use this data to create a treatment plan just for you.

Acquiring Awareness of Triggers and Techniques for Avoidance

To effectively manage rosacea flare-ups, it is essential to identify their triggers. Certain skincare products, sun exposure, hot drinks, spicy foods, alcohol, and stress are common triggers. You can learn more about your symptom causes by keeping a journal. After you've figured out what sets off your skin problems, it's time to start taking steps to prevent them. Sunscreen, mild skin care products, stress reduction tactics, and dietary adjustments can all help.

Creating a Skincare Programme

Skin that is prone to rosacea must adhere to a mild skincare regimen. Face washes with a gentle cleanser and lukewarm water should be done twice a day. After washing, use a soft towel to pat dry. Make sure to moisturize your skin regularly to keep it hydrated. Look for products that are specifically made for sensitive skin. Stay away from abrasive equipment and aggressive exfoliants; they can irritate your skin.

Picking the Right Cosmetics

For delicate skin, look for cosmetics that are fragrance-free and non-comedogenic. Keep an eye out for labels that say they're good for sensitive skin or rosacea. The calming properties of minerals, such as zinc oxide and titanium dioxide, make them a viable option for cosmetics. Before using any new facial product, make sure it works on a small area first.

Dealing with Stress and Promoting Emotional Health

Because stress can bring on flare-ups of rosacea, it is essential to manage stress to keep the condition under control. Deep breathing, yoga, meditation, or just being outside in nature are all great ways to relax. If your mental or emotional health is suffering, it may be helpful to talk to someone, whether that's a friend, family member, or therapist.

Sun Protection and Its Significance

Sun protection is essential for rosacea sufferers because sun exposure can aggravate their symptoms. No matter the weather, always use a broad-spectrum sunscreen that has an SPF of 30 or greater. Protect yourself from the sun by donning a hat and other headgear, and stay indoors during the hottest parts of the day. An additional layer of protection could be provided by a mineral sunscreen that includes titanium dioxide or zinc oxide.

Rosacea Dietary Guidelines

Food and drink do not cause rosacea per se, although they can bring on flare-ups. Foods high in histamine, alcohol, heat, and spicy foods are common triggers. If you want to know what foods set off your symptoms, it could help to keep a food journal. Stick to a healthy eating plan that includes plenty of fresh produce, lean meats, and whole grains.

Making Physical Activity a Part of Your Daily Life

If you suffer from rosacea, it's important to exercise regularly so that your symptoms don't worsen. Try some yoga, swimming, or low-impact walking instead. To prevent flare-ups, exercise in a cool place and stay away from things that make you sweat too much or get too hot.

Keeping Tabs on Symptoms and Development

Journal or keep a diary of your rosacea symptoms, what provokes them, and how your treatment is going. Bear in mind the efficacy of your therapies, any changes to your skin, and any new triggers you may find. To make any necessary adjustments to your treatment plan, share this information with your dermatologist during your follow-up sessions.

Rosacea Support Groups and Other Tools for Patients

Patients suffering from rosacea can benefit greatly from the emotional support, advice, and resources offered by online communities and support groups. By participating in these groups, you can meet others who can relate to your situation and learn from their stories and insights. You can find educational materials, treatment instructions, and support options for rosacea on trustworthy websites and in organizations that focus on the condition.

CHAPTER 5

ROSACEA SKIN CARE

Effortless Methods of Cleaning:

Rosacea sufferers must take extra care when washing their faces so as not to aggravate their skin's sensitivity. When washing sensitive skin, choose a gentle, non-abrasive cleanser. Scrubbing too vigorously or using hot water could bring on an outbreak. To avoid harsh chemicals, wash with lukewarm water and dry with a gentle towel.

Methods for Moisturiser Treatment of Rosacea:

Skin prone to rosacea must be moisturized frequently to keep it hydrated and to fortify its protective barrier. If you want to avoid irritating your skin, use a moisturizer that is not comedogenic and doesn't include any fragrance. Hydrating and soothing the skin without irritating it or blocking its pores are the goals of ingredients like niacinamide, ceramides, and hyaluronic acid.

How to Select Skincare Products That Will Not Irritate:

Choose rosacea skincare products with caution; look for hypoallergenic, non-comedogenic, alcohol-, fragrance-, and harsh preservative-free labels. You can find out if a new product is good for your skin type by applying it to a tiny patch first.

Advice on Choosing and Applying Sunscreen:

Sun protection is essential for rosacea management because prolonged exposure to UV rays can cause flare-ups. Choose a broad-spectrum sunscreen that is developed for sensitive skin and has an SPF of 30 or higher. Use a thick layer of sunscreen and reapply it every two hours, or more frequently if you perspire heavily or are outside.

Tips for Getting Rid of Rosacea with Cosmetics:

For sensitive skin, choose cosmetics products that are either mineral-based or have non-comedogenic formulations. To reduce the appearance of redness, try using a primer or color-correcting lotion with a green tinge. Never use a harsh cleanser to remove heavy or oil-based makeup, and be careful when applying it.

Skincare Regimen for the Night:

Your skin may rejuvenate and heal itself as you sleep if you follow a nocturnal skincare regimen. After cleansing your face with a mild cleanser, apply a calming moisturizer to lock in moisture for the night. To maximize results, think about adding serums or treatments that contain peptides or antioxidants.

A Skincare Emergency Plan for Dealing with Flare-Ups:

Calming and relaxing the skin should be your priority during flare-ups. Apply cold compresses, wash with mild soap, and stay away from hot water to alleviate inflammation. Reduce inflammation and pain using aloe vera gel or an anti-inflammatory medication that includes chamomile or oat extract.

Restoration of the Skin's Barrier Function:

An important part of rosacea management is restoring the skin's protective barrier. For a stronger skin barrier, try using occlusive agents like petrolatum or dimethicone, moisturizers that are high in ceramides, and barrier repair creams. If you want to keep the barrier in good shape, you shouldn't use harsh products or exfoliate too much.

Modern Skincare Procedures:

Advanced skincare treatments might help some people whose rosacea symptoms don't go away permanently. For more choices, such as laser therapy, intense pulsed light (IPL), or prescription drugs like azelaic acid or topical antibiotics, see a dermatologist. Inflammation, redness, and visible blood vessels can all be alleviated with these treatments.

A Few Pointers for Rosacea in Men:

Men who experience rosacea can also benefit from following basic skincare principles, but they should look for products that are lightweight, non-greasy, and absorb fast without leaving any residue. To lessen the risk of irritation, you might want to try shaving using a sensitive skin cream or gel. Choose a calming, fragrance-free aftershave instead of an alcohol-based one.

CHAPTER 6

DEALING WITH ROSACEA CAUSES

Recognizing Individual Resonance

The first step in efficient rosacea management is to identify personal triggers. Because everyone's symptoms are different, it's important to keep track of what makes them worse. Environmental variables, stress, and dietary considerations are all examples of potential triggers.

Avoiding Common Triggers

Several well-known factors can make rosacea symptoms worse. Some examples of these are sun exposure, extreme temperatures, spicy foods, alcohol, and particular skin care products. People can greatly lessen the severity and frequency of flare-ups by learning to identify and stay away from certain triggers.

Weather and Pollution as Environmental Triggers

Rosacea symptoms can be brought on by changes in the weather, including very hot or cold temperatures, strong winds, or high humidity. Air pollution, such as smoke or smog, can exacerbate the symptoms as well. To reduce the impact of these environmental factors, it is important to wear clothes that protect the skin, apply sunscreen regularly, and stay out of the sun for lengthy periods.

What to Avoid on a Diet: Spicy Foods and Alcohol

Some foods and drinks, especially spicy ones and alcohol, might make rosacea worse. For those who suffer from rosacea, it's best to figure out what foods bring on their symptoms and stay away from them whenever feasible. The health of your skin can be improved by eating a balanced diet that is high in fruits, vegetables, and whole grains.

Managing Stress and Emotional Triggers

Rosacea symptoms can be exacerbated by emotional factors like stress. It might be helpful to manage stress by practicing relaxation techniques like yoga, deep breathing exercises, or meditation. Individuals can also benefit from reaching out to loved ones or a therapist for support when dealing with emotional stressors.

Cosmetic and Skincare Triggers

If you have sensitive skin or rosacea, you should avoid using cosmetics and skincare products that include harsh components. To avoid flare-ups, choose mild, non-comedogenic products and stay away from those containing alcohol or scents. It is also recommended to do a patch test on an inconspicuous area before applying a new facial product.

Potential Drug and Therapy Side Effects

Some treatments and drugs, including oral pills and specific topical creams, can cause or worsen rosacea symptoms. To be sure they aren't doing anything to aggravate their rosacea, people should talk to their doctor about their disease.

Ways to Control Triggers in Your Daily Life

Making changes to one's way of life can help a great deal in managing the factors that can provoke rosacea. A regular skincare regimen, daily sunscreen application, enough hydration, sufficient sleep, and avoidance of extreme temperatures are all possible components.

Crafting an Incident Log

If you suffer from rosacea and want to find out what sets your symptoms off, keeping a trigger diary might be a great help. People can keep track of things like their food intake, environmental factors, skincare routine, stress levels, and episodes of flare-ups in the notebook. With this data, we can better identify and stay away from potential dangers.

Methods for Reducing the Risk of Triggers

Finding triggers is just half the battle; you also need to figure out how to lessen your vulnerability to them. Some things you can do to help include taking precautions like wearing a hat and gloves when outside, using a humidifier when it's dry, avoiding hot water, being gentle with your skincare routine, and learning to relax when you're stressed.

Individuals can successfully treat rosacea and enhance the general health and appearance of their skin by utilizing these tactics and recognizing their particular triggers. When dealing with rosacea, it can be helpful to have open lines of communication with healthcare practitioners and skincare specialists.

CHAPTER 7

DEALING WITH THE MENTAL AND EMOTIONAL EFFECTS

Rosacea and Its Emotional Impact:

In addition to the obvious physical effects, rosacea can have a profound psychological impact on those who suffer from it. Experiencing visual symptoms like redness of the face, pimples, and visible blood vessels can often make people feel self-conscious, embarrassed, and even depressed or anxious. People living with rosacea often experience real and normal emotional reactions, and it's important to acknowledge them.

Methods for Dealing with Stress and Anxiety:

Improving rosacea sufferers' general health begins with helping them manage their stress and anxiety. Approaches like yoga or tai chi for relaxation, regular exercise, a balanced diet, and deep breathing exercises can have a significant positive impact. Professional counseling or therapy from a therapist versed in cognitive-behavioral techniques can also help one learn to control anxious thoughts and feelings.

Developing Confidence in One'sself and One's Body:

Managing a noticeable skin condition, such as rosacea, can put a person's self-esteem and body image through their paces. Improving one's self-image can be accomplished by self-care routines, highlighting one's accomplishments and qualities, and rephrasing negative beliefs regarding one's physical appearance. Keep in mind that there are many different kinds of beauty, and rosacea in no way determines a person's value or attractiveness.

A Conversation with a Loved One:

Communicating honestly and openly with loved ones helps build bridges of understanding and support. Make your loved ones more understanding by teaching them about rosacea, what causes it, and how it affects your mental health. When dealing with the emotional components of rosacea, it can be really helpful to have the support and understanding of those closest to you.

Looking into Support Groups and Therapy:

Anxieties can be greatly alleviated by joining rosacea support groups or going to therapy on an individual basis. These groups provide a supportive environment where people may talk about their struggles, learn from others' stories, and get advice from experts. It can be encouraging to connect with people who understand the emotional journey of living with rosacea.

Practices in Mindfulness and Meditation:

Rosacea sufferers can benefit from increased emotional resilience, better stress management, and general well-being through mindfulness and meditation practices. Practices of mindfulness, such as paying attention in the here and now without attaching any value judgments, can help alleviate future worry and poor self-esteem. Emotional well-being can benefit from regular meditation sessions because they bring about relaxation and inner tranquility.

Conquering Social Obstacles:

Having a visible skin condition, such as rosacea, can make social interactions more difficult. You can learn to handle social encounters with more assurance by cultivating coping mechanisms like self-compassion, establishing healthy boundaries, and prioritizing real connections over superficial ones. It's important to keep in mind that true connections are formed through shared interests and personality traits, not just how someone looks.

Establishing Practical Goals:

Maintaining emotional health requires setting reasonable goals for rosacea treatment and control. There may not be a permanent cure for rosacea, therefore it's crucial to realize that controlling symptoms is a continual process and to seek professional guidance when necessary. Reducing the stress and frustration that comes with having high expectations is possible by adopting a realistic perspective.

Raising a Glass to Minor Successes:

Gaining self-assurance and inspiration can be as simple as acknowledging and enjoying minor successes in rosacea management. Every accomplishment is worthy of praise, whether it's an efficient skincare regimen, the management of triggers, or the ability to handle difficult social situations with grace and dignity. To cope with the emotional effects of rosacea, it is helpful to celebrate any progress, no matter how tiny because this encourages more good behavior and builds resilience.

Strategies for Coping in the Long Run and Resilience:

Developing coping mechanisms, cultivating social support, and keeping a good attitude in the face of adversity are all steps in the process of building resilience. Consistent self-care routines, continuous communication with healthcare providers, adaptability to symptom changes, and prioritizing emotional well-being alongside physical health are long-term coping strategies for rosacea. The ability to bounce back from life's inevitable challenges is a key component of resilience training for those living with rosacea.

CHAPTER 8

REDNESS, INFLAMMATION, AND OTHER MEDICAL ISSUES

Heart Health and Rosacea

There is a multi-faceted relationship between rosacea and heart health. Heart conditions including high blood pressure, coronary artery disease, and stroke may be more common in people who suffer from rosacea. Endothelial dysfunction, a consequence of rosacea-related inflammation, compromises blood vessel health and increases the risk of cardiovascular problems.

Topical steroids and oral antibiotics are two examples of rosacea treatments that can be harmful to the cardiovascular system. Developing treatment strategies for patients with rosacea, particularly those with previous cardiovascular diseases, requires healthcare practitioners to carefully examine these issues.

Connections Between Rosacea and Gastrointestinal Disorders

Some gastrointestinal (GI) problems, such as Helicobacter pylori infection or small intestine bacterial overgrowth (SIBO), may be associated with rosacea, according to research. Systemic inflammation, which can be brought on by several illnesses, can make rosacea symptoms worse.

Moreover, treating underlying gastrointestinal disorders has been reported to improve skin health in certain rosacea patients. This highlights the need to address gastrointestinal health as part of a holistic strategy for rosacea management.

Rosacea and Hormonal Discord

Changes in estrogen and androgen levels, in particular, can impact the onset and severity of rosacea. Periods, pregnancies, and menopause are all times of hormonal upheaval that can cause a woman's rosacea symptoms to change.

Treatment regimens for rosacea sufferers can be fine-tuned by considering the effects of hormonal changes on skin health, which can be better understood with an understanding of these impacts.

Emotional Well-being and Rosacea

The effects of rosacea on psychological well-being are substantial. The apparent skin signs of rosacea can cause many people to feel embarrassed, have low self-esteem, and be anxious. Interactions with others, relationships, and general health can all be impacted by this.

Managing the emotional components of rosacea alongside medical treatment might be helped by psychological support, including counseling or therapy. Integral to holistic rosacea management is the treatment of mental health issues.

Lupus and Other Autoimmune Disorders

Even though rosacea isn't an autoimmune illness in and of itself, it can be associated with lupus and rheumatoid arthritis, among others. Inflammation and dysfunction of the immune system are hallmarks of both rosacea and autoimmune disorders.

In evaluating and treating rosacea, particularly in patients with co-occurring autoimmune disorders, healthcare practitioners can benefit from a better understanding of these possible associations.

Sensitivities and Allergies

Rosacea flare-ups can be brought on or worsened by allergies and sensitivities. Some foods, exposure to the sun or high temperatures, skincare products, and medications are common triggers.

The key to effectively controlling rosacea symptoms is identifying and avoiding certain triggers. Individuals who feel that their rosacea is being worse by certain triggers may be advised to undergo allergy testing.

Effects of Rosacea Medications

Rosacea can be affected, for better or worse, by several drugs. To alleviate the redness and swelling caused by rosacea, doctors often recommend anti-inflammatory lotions or topical antibiotics. But rosacea can get worse with long-term use of oral steroids or drugs that widen blood vessels.

Healthcare practitioners must carefully examine their patients' prescription records to identify any possible drug interactions or adverse effects that could impact the management of rosacea.

Handling several Health Issues

Diabetes, high blood pressure, or autoimmune diseases are additional symptoms experienced by many people with rosacea. A multidisciplinary team of healthcare experts is necessary for the management of many chronic diseases.

Treatment programs that take into account the interdependence of various illnesses and put an emphasis on holistic well-being are the result of collaborative care.

Coordinated Methods of Patient Care

Patients with rosacea and other co-occurring conditions benefit from interdisciplinary care teams that work together to meet their unique healthcare requirements. On occasion, this may involve specialists in dermatology, general medicine, gastroenterology, allergies, mental health, and other related fields.

Collaborative care improves treatment results and patient support by encouraging team members to communicate and work together.

Studying the Interactions Between Different Conditions

Rosacea and other health issues have complicated links, which are still being investigated. Research on the connections between rosacea and cardiovascular health, gastrointestinal issues, hormonal effects, autoimmune diseases, allergies, and drug side effects helps fill gaps in our knowledge.

Innovative methods for controlling rosacea and its related health concerns are informed by this research, which also provides evidence-based practices. Improve patient care and results by keeping up with new research.

CHAPTER 9

DEALING WITH ROSACEA EVERY DAY

Travel Advice for Rosacea Patients

Being well-prepared is essential for a nice travel experience with rosacea. Find out as much as you can about the local weather and ecology before you go. Be sure to include the necessary apparel and skincare treatments in case of any weather-related breakouts.

Choose mild, fragrance-free skincare products, including moisturizers and sunscreen with a high sun protection factor (SPF). Touch-ups while on the go may be a breeze with travel-sized products. To protect your face from the sun, think about packing a hat and sunglasses. Staying hydrated will help keep your skin healthy.

Working with Rosacea: Overcoming Professional Obstacles

There may be some special considerations for dealing with rosacea on the job. Keeping an open line of contact with your boss or HR might help. To decrease stigma and increase understanding, educate your coworkers about rosacea.

Take breaks or practice mindfulness throughout the day to deal with stress, which is a typical trigger. For on-the-go skincare touch-ups, keep your necessities in a desk drawer, and if you'd like to wear makeup, look for options that are gentler on sensitive skin.

Rosacea and Love Relationships

Rosacea necessitates self-assurance and open communication to date and sustains relationships. Communicate your situation to your partners as soon as possible. Tell them what rosacea is and how it might impact your daily life and confidence.

Avoid situations that can set off your triggers by opting for indoor dates or places with dim lighting. Make time for self-care a priority and look for traits in a partner beyond how they seem.

Rosacea Treatment for Expectant Mothers

Rosacea might be affected by hormonal changes that occur during pregnancy. To create a skincare regimen that is safe to use throughout pregnancy, talk to your obstetrician and dermatologist. While pregnant, stay away from toxins and medications that aren't safe.

If you see any changes in your skin, be sure to adapt your routine accordingly. To enhance general well-being, it is important to stay hydrated, consume a balanced diet, and manage stress.

Skin Redness and Inflammation in Young People

Problems with social pressures and low self-esteem can exacerbate rosacea in children and teenagers. For advice on the best course of treatment, see a pediatric dermatologist. Instill self-assurance in young people by teaching them about rosacea and how to manage it.

To overcome obstacles connected to self-image, it is important to encourage a good skincare regimen and offer mental support.

Athletes and Physical Fitness

Participating in physical activities that involve rosacea necessitates careful planning. To avoid flushing and overheating, opt for moderately strenuous activity. To keep yourself comfortable, use light, airy clothing made of sweat-wicking materials.

Before going outside, make sure to use sunscreen. To keep cool, think about using cooling towels or sprays. Cool down and stay away from danger by taking breaks when you need them.

Promoting Change and Bringing Attention

To increase knowledge and awareness about rosacea, advocacy is essential. Get involved with advocacy organizations or support groups to meet like-minded people and gain access to resources.

Take part in public awareness campaigns or projects aimed at rosacea education. Inspire others and help dispel the stigma by sharing your story.

Handling Outbursts in Social Contexts

Being well-prepared and practicing self-care techniques are essential for effectively managing social flares. Your dermatologist may recommend a "flare-up kit" that includes calming skincare products, any medicine they prescribe, and, if you like, concealing cosmetics.

To create a nurturing atmosphere, let loved ones know what you need. Learn to relax to control your stress levels and lessen the likelihood of flare-ups.

Rosacea and Ageing: What to Expect and What to Change

Skin changes and new concerns may emerge for rosacea sufferers as they become older. Work with your dermatologist to modify your skincare regimen to combat rosacea and other signs of aging.

Make sure to protect yourself from the sun, stay hydrated, and use moderate skincare products. When dealing with rosacea as you age, it's important to accept yourself as you are and prioritize your health.

Advice on Maintaining Optimism and Strength

When dealing with rosacea, it's important to keep a positive attitude and be resilient. Take time for yourself to do things you enjoy, like meditation, yoga, or a hobby, that help you relax and de-stress.

As you navigate life with rosacea, it's important to surround yourself with people who will support you and understand. Acknowledge and reward yourself for controlling your illness, no matter how small, and always keep in mind that you are more than just your skin.

CHAPTER 10

PROSPECTS FOR ROSACEA STUDIES AND TREATMENTS IN THE FUTURE

Exciting Fields of Study

• The study of Rosacea is progressing in several encouraging directions, including the investigation of its genetic components, the function of the immune system, and the skin microbiota. Research into the routes of inflammation and neurovascular dysregulation is also on the rise, which could lead to new insights into the causes of rosacea.

Recent Developments in Treatment Approaches

There have been great advancements in the treatment of rosacea in recent years. A wide variety of options are becoming available to address various subtypes of rosacea and patient demands, including topical medicines, systemic therapy, lasers, and light-based treatments. These developments highlight the importance of tailored treatment programs for the best results.

Advanced Medical Technology and Rosacea

• Precision-based rosacea treatment takes into account each patient's unique genetic makeup, environmental factors, and disease trajectory when planning a course of treatment. Emphasizing the need for a focused and personalized approach to controlling rosacea, this strategy seeks to maximize therapy efficacy while minimizing unwanted effects.

Initiatives Focusing on the Patient

• Patient-centered care programs in rosacea stress the significance of listening to patients, learning about their desired outcomes, and educating and supporting them as they navigate treatment. Patients are more likely to stick to their treatment regimens and have better results when they have access to information and tools.

The Role of Telemedicine and Technology in Rosacea Treatment

By facilitating remote consultations, monitoring, and support, technology, and telemedicine are revolutionizing rosacea care. Better accessibility, convenience, and continuity of care for rosacea patients are outcomes of increased communication between patients and healthcare professionals made possible by digital tools and platforms.

Cooperation in Rosacea Studies

Advancements and information exchange in rosacea research are propelled by collaborative endeavors among researchers, doctors, industry associates, and patient advocacy organizations. In the end, everyone dealing with rosacea benefits from multidisciplinary cooperation since it increases our knowledge of the disease's pathogenesis, treatment options, and patient outcomes.

Supporting Patients and Involving the Community

• Community involvement programs and patient advocacy groups are crucial in bringing attention to rosacea, offering support, and fighting for better treatment options. These initiatives encourage learning, lessen discrimination, and give people a voice in their healthcare choices.

Worldwide Campaigns to Raise Rosacea Awareness

• The significance of early diagnosis and therapy of rosacea, as well as its effects on quality of life, are being brought to the attention of the public through worldwide campaigns. The global community can benefit from more accurate knowledge about rosacea thanks to collaborative initiatives, educational materials, and outreach programs.

Possible Solutions and Future Prospects

• A permanent solution to the rosacea problem is still out of reach, but new developments in the field give promise for better long-term management and symptom control. Future treatments for rosacea may be more effective if we learn more about its biological basis, develop preventative measures, and use targeted therapeutics.

Backing Rosacea Research and New Approaches

• Funding efforts, encouraging scientific collaboration, and lobbying for legislation that prioritizes dermatological research are ways to support rosacea research and innovation. If we want to make a difference and provide better treatment for people with rosacea, we must invest in research facilities, clinical trials, and educational programs.

The ongoing endeavors to improve outcomes and quality of life for persons impacted by rosacea are exemplified by these domains, which together provide a holistic strategy for rosacea research, treatment, and advocacy.

9 798333 850607